Distribution, publication, and copying in any form are prohibited and subject to damages.

TEN HYPNOSES

Copying, publishing, and sharing with third parties are only permitted with the written consent of the author. Please observe the notes on copyright and usage.

Distribution, publication, and copying in any form are prohibited and subject to damages.

Copying, publishing, and sharing with third parties are only permitted with the written consent of the author. Please observe the notes on copyright and usage.

Distribution, publication, and copying in any form are prohibited and subject to damages.

Ingo Michael Simon

TEN HYPNOSES

40

OVERCOMING RESENTMENT AND ANGER

Copying, publishing, and sharing with third parties are only permitted with the written consent of the author. Please observe the notes on copyright and usage.

Distribution, publication, and copying in any form are prohibited and subject to damages.

© 2024 Ingo Michael Simon
All rights reserved.
Independently published
www.ingosimon.com

Important Notes for Urgent Attention:

The contents of this book are based on the practical experiences of the author with hypnosis applications and psychotherapy in a trance state. Although the author has strived for the utmost care, errors or misunderstandings in the presentation cannot be completely excluded. Therapeutic work with people and the application of hypnosis are solely the responsibility of the hypnotist. It cannot be ruled out that parts of this book may be misunderstood or that the application of a presented procedure may cause an undesirable reaction in the client. The author also assumes no co-responsibility if work with a client is carried out with reference to the statements in this book.

The Author:

Ingo Michael Simon studied psychology and education and is a hypnotherapist with practices in southwestern Germany and Switzerland. With the help of hypnosis-supported psychotherapy, he primarily treats people with persistent psychological conditions. His practice focuses on anxiety disorders, pathological compulsions, and psychosomatic illnesses. His therapeutic offerings mainly include classical and modern hypnosis applications and the dreamland therapy he developed himself.

Copying, publishing, and sharing with third parties are only permitted with the written consent of the author. Please observe the notes on copyright and usage.

Distribution, publication, and copying in any form are prohibited and subject to damages.

INTRODUCTION	6
COPYRIGHT AND USAGE	8
HYPNOSIS 1	10
HYPNOSIS 2	16
HYPNOSIS 3	22
HYPNOSIS 4	28
HYPNOSIS 5	38
HYPNOSIS 6	44
HYPNOSIS 7	51
HYPNOSIS 8	56
HYPNOSIS 9	61
HYPNOSIS 10	67
ALL TITLES IN THE SERIES	74

Copying, publishing, and sharing with third parties are only permitted with the written consent of the author. Please observe the notes on copyright and usage.

Introduction

The series "Ten Hypnoses" is very well known in Germany, Austria, and Switzerland as a collection of texts for therapeutic work and is used by numerous psychotherapeutic practices, doctors, therapists, coaches, and other helping professionals. I am pleased to now be able to offer these texts in other countries as well.

Most therapists have their own methods for inducing and deepening trance as well as for exiting trance. Therefore, I have focused on the main part of the hypnosis. The texts in this book can be integrated as the main part into any hypnosis process. The texts in this collection use various hypnosis techniques. I will not explain these in detail, as I assume that users have the appropriate training. It is also not necessary to understand the exact structure or functioning of the different parts. The texts can simply be read aloud, and they will have their effect.

Decide for yourself which text best suits your client or patient at any given time. You can also combine passages from different texts. It is not about using all ten hypnoses in sequence. It is a selection of possibilities.

I want to emphasize that books cannot replace therapy. Psychotherapy or other therapeutic treatments involve much more. A careful diagnosis is the necessary basis for deciding on the use of methods, including whether hypnosis or one of my texts should be used. Even in this case, preparatory discussions, follow-up discussions during the session, and of course, a therapeutic concept for the sequence of sessions and the content approaches are essential parts of therapy. This cannot and should not be achieved with a collection of texts.

In any case, I wish you much success in your work and I am pleased if my text templates can contribute in a small way.

Ingo Michael Simon

Copyright and Usage

Copying, publishing, and sharing with third parties is prohibited and only permitted with the written consent of the author. Please observe the following copyright and usage guidelines.

This work has been carefully crafted and created to the best of the author's knowledge and personal experience. It comprises text templates and application guidelines for professional hypnosis sessions. The author is a licensed psychotherapist with extensive experience in psychotherapy, coaching, and personal training using hypnotic techniques and methods. Nevertheless, the author and the publisher assume no liability for the accuracy of information, instructions, and advice, nor for any typographical errors. The author and publisher accept no responsibility or liability for the application of these texts and recommendations with clients or patients, nor for any potential consequences or unexpected reactions. It is expressly noted that the application of therapeutic and advisory techniques and formulations lies solely and entirely within the responsibility of the practitioner. This also applies to adherence to the boundaries of legally regulated medical and therapeutic practices. The fact that a book containing action proposals is freely available for sale does not imply that its application with clients or patients is permitted for everyone.

Hypnosis 1

... ... You have felt a deep sense of resentment and anger for years now ... ... It has become, maybe for a long time now, a kind of underlying feeling that is always there ... ... You notice it because you are always somewhat grumpy, and you've built a real wall around yourself ... ... You may not have always noticed it yourself, but you've experienced others telling you about it ... ... and that you've become more and more distant ... ... When you look back, you can see that many people have pulled away ... ... just like you have ... ... because your grumpy mood doesn't exactly invite small talk ... ... You know this, and you ask yourself why it's like this ... ... Of course, you also know what has made you so fundamentally angry, at least you know part of it ... ... Maybe you'd say that it's the injustices of life or the actions of harmful people that have worn you down ... ... And you're right, but there's more to it ... ... There's always more, because why else would you direct your anger towards those who are not involved or even towards yourself? ... ... We often do that ... ... we take our frustrations out on the next person who talks to us ... ... but those are usually brief moments or exceptions ... ... Exceptions, because we're not constantly frustrated ... ... Neither are you, but somehow it has come to be that a certain underlying frustration just hasn't gone away ... ... You ask yourself what's really going on ... ... and you've blamed yourself a lot ... ... Now it's time to stop blaming yourself, or at least put it on hold, so you can breathe again and deal with your anger without building a wall ... ... Let's work together on freeing you, because it's possible ... ... You can change all of this ... ...

... ... A lot has happened in your life, even more than you can spontaneously recall now ... ... There are always events that shape and influence us that we don't directly perceive ... ... some we never find out about ... ... But when you experienced humiliations and defeats in the past, you could have used some help ... ... Maybe many of those humiliations or defeats couldn't have been avoided, but it could have helped if someone had comforted you ... ... Comfort and care could have helped a lot ... ... Love could have helped ... ... because comfort and love catch us when we fall ... ... Comfort and love reach out to us when we're down ... ... If there had been someone who told you that you were still a valuable person or that they liked or loved you, you would have been able to feel your self-worth better … … Maybe there was no one who could or wanted to tell you that … … or maybe they just couldn't reach you properly … … Perhaps your trust was so deeply shaken that you couldn't imagine it anymore … … Today, you are here, and in this trance, you are close to yourself … … Whatever is going on out there, you are close to yourself in your feelings now, and you can give yourself this comfort … … as much and as lovingly as is possible now … … Even the peace of this trance and the soothing words you hear can give you comfort if you are ready to hear and feel it … … [about 20 seconds of silence] … …

+++ Variant 1: Anger, General +++

… … There is a way to deal with your feelings and the experiences of the past … … You have found someone to talk to, not only in our contact, but also within yourself … … You've probably often talked or negotiated with yourself, maybe even struggled … … in your thoughts or in your feelings … … But now you have a new way of connecting with yourself ... ... In the state of trance, you can reach all your feelings, especially those that you don't notice so well in everyday life ... ... that's why in trance, you can repeatedly engage in a helpful dialogue with yourself ... ... and then you can also make a decision ... ... So you decide, on the one hand, to finally process the feelings of the past completely, because you know you are not alone with them ... ... and on the other hand, you decide to allow beautiful feelings again and to give life a chance ... ... to give encounters with people a chance and to meet them freely and openly ... ... You, therefore, carefully and mindfully pay attention to openness and freedom within yourself ... ... and you push the anger aside, even and especially if you find pain and many tears behind it ... ... You free them and feel comfort and support in the process ... ... [about 30 seconds of silence] ... ...

+++ End of Variant 1 +++

+++ Variant 2: Anger as Self-Aggression +++

... ... There is a way to deal with your feelings and the experiences of the past ... ... You have found someone to talk to, not only in our contact, but also within yourself ... ... You've probably often talked or negotiated with yourself, maybe even struggled ... ... you've judged yourself and turned your anger inward ... ... But now you have a new way of connecting with yourself ... ... that's why you can re-enter a helpful dialogue with yourself and then make a decision ... ... So you decide, on the one hand, to finally process the feelings of the past completely, because you know you are not alone with them ... ... and on the other hand, you decide to make peace with yourself and finally forgive yourself ... ... whatever you have been blaming yourself for ... ... You want to, and you are allowed to be there for yourself now ... ... and you push the anger aside, even and especially if you find pain and many tears behind it ... ... You free them and feel comfort and support in the process ... ... You even rediscover self-love ... ... [about 20 seconds of silence] ... ...

+++ End of Variant 2 +++

... ... Now, rest ... ... Simply stay in your feeling and let your body's relaxation become a deep inner relaxation ... ...

You are close to yourself, and you are safe ... ... There are no humiliations and no defeats here ... ... The painful feelings you experience have been with you for a long time ... ... You are processing them internally right now, and it hurts ... ... But the pain will soon fade, and you'll realize that you have truly processed the past ... ... Then you'll feel more and more that you are carried by comfort and self-love now and every day ... ... and anger really dissolves ... ... and you feel freer and lighter ... ... more content and happier ... ... every day freer and lighter ... ... every day more content and happier ... ...

Hypnosis 2

... ... You seek freedom from the old and long-lasting anger; you want to finally experience freedom again ... ... This freedom is possible, and even more ... ... You can reactivate a completely different sense of life ... ... a free and constructive sense of life, characterized by curiosity and openness ... ... This feeling is still there; it has always been there ... ... and as soon as the anger subsides, you will rediscover this good sense of life ... ... There is a place where all of this is possible ... ... Far away from all burdens, far away from anger and pain, there is this very special land ... ... the land of dreams ... ... It lies somewhere within you and, at the same time, far away and very close ... ... You are going there now; you are already there ... ...

... ... You stand in the middle of a forest, on a wide path ... ... You start walking, and your path leads you deeper and deeper into this forest, which is the forest of your own thoughts ... ... and each tree represents a thought ... ... There are melancholic and sad thoughts within you ... ... Failures and disappointments that have made you sad ... ...

There are thoughts and memories of relationships that have broken, of people who have left the shared path with you ... ... or you ended it yourself and took a new path, perhaps disappointed and hurt and full of sad anger ... ... Anger that eventually turned into a deep resentment ... ... And there are other thoughts that stand here as trees in this forest because every thought remains as a memory in the land of dreams ... ... nothing is ever truly forgotten because what has happened has happened and is and remains a part of your story ... ... You recognize your own memories and thoughts as you go deeper into the forest ... ... deeper into trance ... ... deeper into your feelings ... ...

... ... You discover the entrance to a cave ... ... At the entrance to the cave is a sign with the inscription ... ... Cave of Uncried Tears ... ... You go inside ... ... It's a stalactite cave, with water dripping from the ceiling and walls ... ... You go deeper and deeper inside and feel that these are your own tears running down the walls ... ... All the tears behind the anger ... ... all the tears you have held back ... ... all the uncried tears ... ... You go deeper and deeper into this cave and feel more and more clearly the emotion hiding behind your anger because here you are in the Cave of

Tears, the Cave of Sadness ... ... Perhaps it is a deep grief that you can feel here ... ... perhaps a loss ... ... possibly despair ... ... Behind the anger, you find in the Cave of Uncried Tears the very emotion that you carry deep within you, the one that has only used anger as a front to remain hidden ... ... But here, in the land of dreams, you see everything very clearly ... ... You feel this emotion within you ... ... You reach the very depth of the cave, in a large chamber, where the emotion you have found becomes very intense ... ... You stand still and let the feeling be fully present ... ... even if it is painful ... ... You are standing in this feeling now ... ... It surrounds you completely ... ... You recognize the feeling behind your anger ... ... [A minute of silence] ... ...

+++ Variant 1: Anger, General +++

... ... You suddenly recognize this particular feeling, and it doesn't really matter why it was there and is there ... ... What's more important now is that you recognize what feeling is really there, whether it is sadness, loneliness, or something else ... ... It was never really about anger ... ...

Anger was just what was expressed outwardly ... ... Anger was just the wall behind which you hid ... ... and far behind the wall, deep in the cave, is the real feeling that you are now experiencing ... ... and you let it be ... ... You feel it, and even if it hurts, it will not harm you ... ... Feelings ... ... honest feelings will never harm you ... ... What can harm you are judgments ... ... Judgments about your feelings, whether they are judged by others or by yourself ... ... Any feeling that you allow and accept, you feel deeply, and then it lets you go ... ... then it becomes a memory and an experience, and that's exactly what is happening right now ... ... and anger fades because you don't need it anymore ... ... Anger dissolves because the wall is no longer necessary; it no longer serves any purpose ... ... You are freeing yourself now, letting all the tears out ... ... [about 20 seconds of silence] ... ...

+++ End of Variant 1 +++

+++ Variant 2: Anger as Self-Aggression +++

... ... You suddenly recognize this particular feeling, and it doesn't really matter why it was there and is there ... ...

What's more important now is that you recognize what feeling is really there, whether it is sadness, loneliness, or something else ... ... It was never really about anger towards yourself or self-destruction ... ... Anger was just what you used to accuse yourself ... ... Anger was just the weapon you had turned against yourself ... ... and far behind the aggression towards yourself, deep in the cave, is the real feeling that you are now experiencing ... ... and you let it be ... ... You feel it, and even if it hurts, it will not harm you ... ... Feelings ... ... honest feelings will never harm you ... ... What can harm you are judgments ... ... Judgments about your feelings and self-punishments through anger ... ... Any feeling that you allow and accept, you feel deeply, and then it lets you go ... ... then it becomes a memory and an experience, and that's exactly what is happening right now ... ... and anger fades because you don't need it anymore ... ... Anger dissolves because the wall is no longer necessary; it no longer serves any purpose ... ... You are freeing yourself now, letting all the tears out ... ... [about 20 seconds of silence] ... ...

+++ End of Variant 2 +++

… … Then the tears stop … … You feel freer and lighter, and you discover an exit … … You see light through the wall of the cave and find an exit … … With a big step, you go out of the cave and back into the forest … … and in this forest of your own thoughts, you find a new path … … one you've never taken before … … It leads you to yourself … … It leads you to peace and freedom … … So you continue on this path of peace … … step by step … … and you think about how the land of dreams is always open to you and always holds a healing path for you … … You can reach the land of dreams very easily … … a part of you is always there … … because the land of dreams is deep within you … … It has always been there … … I'm just telling you about it … …

Hypnosis 3

… … You've experienced many defeats and humiliations … … Many things have hit you hard, and some blows have hit you much harder than you expected … … This has made you angry and grumpy, but you want to feel good again … … and to do this, you've chosen the path of trance … … So, you've recognized … … Hypnosis is a very special path … …

… … If you know the principle of hypnosis, you also know … … Suggestions heard in hypnosis work especially quickly … … and … … you will experience this effect … … if you can truly embrace hypnosis … … because you are using the rapid effect of hypnosis for yourself … … You want to let go of resentment and anger … … you want to overcome the feeling of inferiority and trust again … …

… … And if this hypnosis succeeds in doing just that, then you are safe … … This hypnosis frees you … … So, this hypnosis can indeed be the first big step … … And because every renewal begins with the first step, we can say … … This is the first step into a free feeling of life … … Maybe you are already eagerly awaiting the effect of hypnosis, or …

... You can already feel the trance, and ... ... you quickly feel the effect of the following suggestions ... ...

... ... Hypnosis opens up a whole new access to your deep feelings, to your unconscious ... ... You can speak with your subconscious ... ... but only in a comfortable and good trance ... ...

... ... Feel your body and notice how calm it feels ... ... Maybe you already feel a very pleasant relaxation ... ... If you can feel relaxation, and you have been relaxing for some time now, then you also feel ... ... The healing connection to your subconscious is already working ... ... or ... ... You will feel it even more intensely in a few moments ... ... when you feel that relaxation ... ...

... ... If you had one wish, you might say ... ... Every feeling of anger and resentment should dissolve ... ... or you might say ... ... Your subconscious can and should help you ... ... or ... ... Every feeling of inferiority should come to an end ... ... and if the wish comes true, then you would know ... ... Now the way is clear for a new sense of life ... ...

+++ Variant 1: Anger, General +++

… … If you imagine self-esteem as a path that you can freely choose, then you can imagine … … You simply walk directly towards strong self-esteem … … You walk towards your self-esteem and thus also towards a good sense of life … … Just imagine it as a path … …

… … And if you can find yourself very quickly on such an inner path, then you probably think … … Good self-esteem is easy to find within … … and … … You can really feel your self-worth … … … Maybe it's only that simple in your imagination and actually takes longer, but if in a few moments you could feel yourself as very valuable, then you would be sure … … Today, you have truly succeeded … once again in feeling good self-esteem and thereby letting go of resentment and anger … … Today it will succeed for sure … maybe also … to overcome all humiliations in this new feeling … … either … … It succeeds right now … … or … … It succeeds at the right time … … who knows … …

… … Everyone experiences this at their own pace … … If you feel during this hypnosis that you are closer to yourself, then at least for you, it is certain … … This hypnosis brings you to yourself … because … You realize that you are a valuable person … …

+++ End of Variant 1 +++

+++ Variant 2: Anger as Self-Aggression +++

... ... If you imagine self-esteem as a path that you can freely choose, then you can imagine ... ... You simply walk directly towards your self-love ... ... You walk towards your self-love and thus also towards a good sense of life ... ... Just imagine it as a path ... ...

... ... And if you can find yourself very quickly on such an inner path, then you probably think ... ... Liberating self-love is easy to find within ... ... and ... ... You can really feel your self-worth in love ... ... Maybe it's only that simple in your imagination and actually takes longer, but if in a few moments you could feel self-love clearly, then you would be sure ... ... Today, you have truly succeeded ... in feeling real self-love and thereby letting go of anger towards yourself ... ... Today it will succeed for sure ... maybe also ... to overcome all humiliations in this new feeling ... ... either ... ... It succeeds right now ... ... or ... ... It succeeds at the right time ... ... who knows ... ...

... ... Everyone experiences this at their own pace ... ... If you feel during this hypnosis that you are closer to yourself, then at least for you, it is certain ... ... This hypnosis brings you to yourself ... because ... You realize that you can accept and even love yourself ... ...

+++ End of Variant 2 +++

... ... When the effect of this trance fully unfolds, the old anger disappears, and your self-esteem becomes stronger, your self-respect and self-love grow ... ... As soon as the full effect sets in, you feel ... ... You are full of self-respect and let go of resentment and anger once and for all ... ... In this trance, you are calm and relaxed and can let go of everything better, and there is an additional, very special feeling ... ... You feel free and light ... now, in this hypnosis ... It is a feeling of inner freedom ... ... It is a feeling of inner recognition and self-respect ... ... that you can perhaps already feel quite well in this hypnosis ... ...

... ... If you consciously perceive your feeling at this moment, then maybe it's already so that ... ... you clearly feel self-love ... ... and ... ... You truly feel relief and inner peace ... ... But even if it takes some time, you can trust because ... ... With each day, you feel your self-love and self-worth more and more ... ... if you trust this hypnosis ... ... Then, you will soon realize ... ... This hypnosis completely dissolves resentment and anger ... ... But all paths are individual and unique ... ... You will find your good path ... ... in your own feelings ... ... So, a new and free sense of life is possible ... ...

Hypnosis 4

… … Offenses and humiliations are painful … … You've experienced that, and it wasn't an easy time … … But now it's time to experience inner and outer freedom again … … to let go of deep resentment because life is very different today … … You can, and you will free yourself … … free yourself from the burden of the past and from the anger … … You can feel good again … … Maybe you know how that works … … or you have an idea of it … … You are certainly convinced of the effect of hypnosis and know that hypnosis can be a path to liberation and a new beginning … … that's why you chose hypnosis … … So, simply pay attention to my voice … … that's all that matters … … and suddenly, everything sounds so familiar … … Everything sounds so coherent and fitting … … and that's exactly why your subconscious is particularly helpful to you today … …

… Hypnosis … is a very special path … [5-10 seconds pause] …

… Suggestions … in hypnosis … work especially quickly … [5-10 seconds pause] …

... You experience this effect ... today ... [5-10 seconds pause] ...

... You want ... to let go of resentment and anger today ... [5-10 seconds pause] ...

... This hypnosis is the first step ... into a new feeling of life ... [5-10 seconds pause] ...

... You feel the effect ... of the following suggestions ... [5-10 seconds pause] ...

... Hypnosis ... is a very special path ... [5-10 seconds pause] ...

... Suggestions ... in hypnosis ... work especially quickly ... [5-10 seconds pause] ...

... You experience this effect ... today ... [5-10 seconds pause] ...

... You want ... to let go of resentment and anger today ... [5-10 seconds pause] ...

... This hypnosis is the first step ... into a new feeling of life ... [5-10 seconds pause] ...

... You feel the effect ... of the following suggestions ... [5-10 seconds pause] ...

... You can ... speak with your subconscious ... [5-10 seconds pause] ...

... The healing connection ... to your subconscious is working ... [5-10 seconds pause] ...

... You feel it in a few moments ... even more intensely ... [5-10 seconds pause] ...

... Your subconscious can ... and should help you now ... [5-10 seconds pause] ...

... Every feeling ... of resentment and anger should now dissolve ... [5-10 seconds pause] ...

... Now the way is clear for a ... new feeling of life ... [5-10 seconds pause] ...

... You can ... speak with your subconscious ... [5-10 seconds pause] ...

... The healing connection ... to your subconscious is working ... [5-10 seconds pause] ...

... You feel it in a few moments ... even more intensely ... [5-10 seconds pause] ...

... Your subconscious can ... and should help you now ... [5-10 seconds pause] ...

... Every feeling ... of resentment and anger should now dissolve ... [5-10 seconds pause] ...

... Now the way is clear for a ... new feeling of life ... [5-10 seconds pause] ...

+++ Variant 1: Anger, General +++

... You walk directly towards a ... strong sense of self-worth ... [5-10 seconds pause] ...

... You walk towards a ... good feeling of life ... [5-10 seconds pause] ...

... Good self-esteem is easy to find ... within ... [5-10 seconds pause] ...

... You can really feel your ... self-worth ... [5-10 seconds pause] ...

... Today it will succeed ... for sure ... [5-10 seconds pause] ...

... It succeeds ... right now ... [5-10 seconds pause] ...

... It succeeds ... at the right time ... [5-10 seconds pause] ...

... This hypnosis brings you to ... yourself ... [5-10 seconds pause] ...

... You recognize that you are a valuable person ... [5-10 seconds pause] ...

... You walk directly towards a ... strong sense of self-worth ... [5-10 seconds pause] ...

... You walk towards a ... good feeling of life ... [5-10 seconds pause] ...

... Good self-esteem is easy to find ... within ... [5-10 seconds pause] ...

... You can really feel your ... self-worth ... [5-10 seconds pause] ...

... Today it will succeed ... for sure ... [5-10 seconds pause] ...

... It succeeds ... right now ... [5-10 seconds pause] ...

... It succeeds ... at the right time ... [5-10 seconds pause] ...

... This hypnosis brings you to ... yourself ... [5-10 seconds pause] ...

... You recognize that you are a valuable person ... [5-10 seconds pause] ...

+++ End of Variant 1 +++

+++ Variant 2: Anger as Self-Aggression +++

... You walk ... directly ... and assertively towards your self-love ... [5-10 seconds pause] ...

... And thus also towards ... a free and good feeling of life ... [5-10 seconds pause] ...

... Good self-esteem is easy to find ... within ... [5-10 seconds pause] ...

... Liberating self-love is easy to find ... within ... [5-10 seconds pause] ...

... You can really feel ... self-love ... [5-10 seconds pause] ...

... Today it will succeed ... for sure ... [5-10 seconds pause] ...

... It succeeds ... right now ... [5-10 seconds pause] ...

... It succeeds ... at the right time ... [5-10 seconds pause] ...

... You recognize ... that you can accept yourself ... [5-10 seconds pause] ...

... You walk ... directly ... and assertively towards your self-love ... [5-10 seconds pause] ...

... And thus also towards ... a free and good feeling of life ... [5-10 seconds pause] ...

... Good self-esteem is easy to find ... within ... [5-10 seconds pause] ...

... Liberating self-love is easy to find ... within ... [5-10 seconds pause] ...

... You can really feel ... self-love ... [5-10 seconds pause] ...

... Today it will succeed ... for sure ... [5-10 seconds pause] ...

... It succeeds ... right now ... [5-10 seconds pause] ...

... It succeeds ... at the right time ... [5-10 seconds pause] ...

... You recognize ... that you can accept yourself ... [5-10 seconds pause] ...

+++ End of Variant 2 +++

... You are ... full of self-respect ... and let go of resentment and anger ... [5-10 seconds pause] ...

... You feel free and ... light ... [5-10 seconds pause] ...

... It is a feeling of ... inner freedom ... [5-10 seconds pause] ...

... It is a feeling of ... inner recognition ... and self-respect ... [5-10 seconds pause] ...

... You truly feel relief and ... inner peace ... [5-10 seconds pause] ...

... With each day, you feel self-love and ... self-worth more strongly ... [5-10 seconds pause] ...

... This hypnosis ... completely dissolves resentment and anger ... [5-10 seconds pause] ...

... You find your ... good path ... [5-10 seconds pause] ...

... So, a ... new feeling of life ... is possible ... [5-10 seconds pause] ...

... You are ... full of self-respect ... and let go of resentment and anger ... [5-10 seconds pause] ...

... You feel free and ... light ... [5-10 seconds pause] ...

... It is a feeling of ... inner freedom ... [5-10 seconds pause] ...

... It is a feeling of ... inner recognition ... and self-respect ... [5-10 seconds pause] ...

... You truly feel relief and ... inner peace ... [5-10 seconds pause] ...

... With each day, you feel self-love and ... self-worth more strongly ... [5-10 seconds pause] ...

... This hypnosis ... completely dissolves resentment and anger ... [5-10 seconds pause] ...

... You find your ... good path ... [5-10 seconds pause] ...

... So, a ... new feeling of life ... is possible ... [5-10 seconds pause] ...

Hypnosis 5

... ... You've decided to close the chapter of past anger and resentment ... ... because you know that only then can you be free ... ...

... ... You've decided to close the chapter of past anger and resentment ... ... because you know you can't change what has already happened ... ...

... ... You've decided to close the chapter of past anger and resentment ... ... because you know that you have learned from all the events and experiences in life ... ...

... ... You've decided to close the chapter of past anger and resentment ... ... because you know that you can start fresh here and now and every day ... ...

+++ Variant 1: Anger, General +++

... ... You finally separate yourself from old patterns of anger and resentment ... ... and that's why you can close the chapter on the past today ... ...

... ... You finally separate yourself from old patterns of anger and resentment ... ... and that's why you can overcome accusations and judgmental attitudes ... ...

... ... You finally separate yourself from old patterns of anger and resentment ... ... and that's why you can use everything from the past as experience ... ...

... ... You finally separate yourself from old patterns of anger and resentment ... ... and that's why you can fully concentrate on the present and feel free ... ...

... ... This is your new beginning in peace and freedom ... ...

+++ End of Variant 1 +++

+++ Variant 2: Resentment and Anger as Self-Aggression +++

... ... You release your feelings and make peace with yourself ... ... and that's why you can close the chapter on the past today ... ...

… … You release your feelings and make peace with yourself … … and that's why you can overcome accusations and judgmental attitudes … …

… … You release your feelings and make peace with yourself … … and that's why you can use everything from the past as experience … …

… … You release your feelings and make peace with yourself … … and that's why you can fully concentrate on the present and feel free … …

… … This is your new beginning in peace and freedom … …

+++ End of Variant 2 +++

… … The relaxation of your body helps you feel inner peace … … because you know that body, mind, and soul are connected … …

… … The relaxation of your body helps you feel inner peace … … because you know that inner freedom is what you need most … …

... ... The relaxation of your body helps you feel inner peace ... ... because you know that what has passed is already done ... ...

... ... The relaxation of your body helps you feel inner peace ... ... because you know that it is truly valuable to look forward and start anew ... ...

... ... This is your new beginning in peace and freedom ... ...

... ... Now, fully immerse yourself in the calm feeling of the moment ... ... because the present moment is always the most important moment in life ... ...

... ... Now, fully immerse yourself in the calm feeling of the moment ... ... because the present is the most important time for you ... ...

... ... Now, fully immerse yourself in the calm feeling of the moment ... ... because only in this way can you keep letting go of the past ... ...

... ... Now, fully immerse yourself in the calm feeling of the moment ... ... because only in this way can you keep shaping each new day ... ...

... ... This is your new beginning in peace and freedom ... ...

... ... You now focus on your ability for peaceful conflict resolution and constructive engagement ... ... because in this way, you let go of the past ... ...

... ... You now focus on your ability for peaceful conflict resolution and constructive engagement ... ... because in this way, you deal with the present, which is what matters ... ...

... ... You now focus on your ability for peaceful conflict resolution and constructive engagement ... ... because in this way, you turn your experience into something good ... ...

... ... You now focus on your ability for peaceful conflict resolution and constructive engagement ... ... because in this way, every day becomes a constructive new beginning ... ...

... ... This is your new beginning in peace and freedom ... ...

... ... Today, you have let go of anger and resentment, and you keep letting go of anger and resentment ... ... and then you move forward with a sense of freedom ... ...

... ... Today, you have let go of anger and resentment, and you keep letting go of anger and resentment ... ... and that's why you can also approach life and people with kindness and openness again ... ...

... ... Today, you have let go of anger and resentment, and you keep letting go of anger and resentment ... ... Yes, you live in the present, because that's what matters ... ... Only the present matters ... ...

Hypnosis 6

… … You have experienced many offenses and humiliations, and all of that has made you angry and distrustful … … and sensitive, because every humiliation, every degradation hurts … … You know you can't change the past … … But you also know that today, you can handle it differently … … that you can let go of the past and, with it, the anger … … At least you can let go of the pain from past offenses and defeats, give them to the past … … and that is the most important thing … … As a memory and experience, you can and will keep the time of offenses and defeats, and that is also important … … because your memories and experiences help you protect yourself better … … to protect yourself without the wall of anger … … to be stronger and to recognize your self-worth … … more than that … … You can process the painful feelings and thus become free again … … You will take care of that today … … in a very special encounter … …

… … Deep within yourself, in the world of your feelings, there is a place of encounter … … a place where you always feel safe and can help yourself ... ... To get there, focus on the feeling in your body ... ... Imagine sinking into the feeling of your body, going deep inside ... ... into your inner center ... ... In fact, you are already there, you just have to recognize it ... ... and there, you let it become quieter and quieter, because you are sinking deeper and deeper into your own feelings ... ... Everything becomes still inside, because everything outside is now meaningless ... ... You feel only inward ... ... You let yourself sink deeper ... ... Now, just listen to my words ... ... Enjoy the silence and just listen to my words ... ... And then you also recognize that there is a special place there in the silence ... ... a place that is just for you ... ... This is the place of inner encounter ... ... and here you feel the pleasant closeness of a very familiar person who gives you security and accompanies you ... ... [About 30 seconds pause] ... ...

... ... You are now encountering yourself within ... ... because there is an experienced and self-confident part of you ... ... because self-confidence and experience are always found deep in your feelings ... ... so also now ... ... So, it is an inner self-encounter ... ... here and now, because this part of you brings a strong sense of self-worth ... ... This part of you knows and feels that you can truly free yourself from resentment and anger ... ... You yourself are there to help ... ... like a friend who you are to yourself today ... ... today and every coming day ... ... Now you are your own helper ... ... You greet yourself with a peaceful and honest embrace ... ... with a positive and pleasant feeling that you can feel in your body if you now pay close attention to your body feeling ... ... You feel this warmth and feel the connection to yourself ... ... to this helper inside you ... ...

+++ Variant 1: Anger, General +++

... ... You remember a situation where you were inferior to another person or a system, an organization, and couldn't do anything about it, even though you were in the right ... ... You remember the pain of the humiliation ... ... You think about why this experience made you so angry and why you built up this wall of anger against everyone ... ... even against those not involved ... ... You wanted to preserve a good feeling of life, and maybe you were once primarily angry at the perpetrators of the past injustice ... ... But your former powerlessness made you angry at everything and everyone ... ... You wonder how it got to the point where anger could dominate your entire feeling of life ... ... You probably know some answers to this question, but not all ... ... So, you ask your helper what he/she knows about it ... ... and this experienced part of you looks at you kindly ... ... now sends you thoughts and feelings or even speaks to you ... ... You now hear deep in the silence a new answer ... ... Just listen and feel what he/she now tells you about yourself ... ... [Please allow about 30 seconds of silence now] ... ...

+++ End of Variant 1 +++

+++ Variant 2: Anger as Self-Aggression +++

... ... You remember a situation where you were inferior to another person or a system, an organization, and couldn't do anything about it, even though you were in the right ... ... You remember the pain of the humiliation ... ... You think about why this experience made you so angry and why you turned the power and aggression of your anger even against yourself ... ... Maybe you thought you had made mistakes or you couldn't forgive yourself for not being able to defend yourself properly ... ... Somehow, you kept blaming yourself, maybe also because your accusations and complaints didn't work outwardly ... ... You may have stopped fighting and then fought against yourself ... ... So, you ask yourself once again how it could have come to the point where anger could dominate your entire feeling of life and turn against yourself ... ... You probably know some answers to this question, but not all ... ... So, you ask your helper what he/she knows about it ... ... and this experienced part of you looks at you kindly ... ... now sends you thoughts and feelings or even speaks to you ... ... You now hear deep in the silence a new answer ... ... Just listen and feel what he/she now tells you about yourself ... ... [Please allow about 30 seconds of silence now] ... ...

+++ End of Variant 2 +++

... ... Pay attention to what is being conveyed to you, and just accept it ... ... Maybe you hear your inner voice ... ... or you have a special thought that you didn't expect ... ... or it is a feeling that suddenly appears ... ... a thought or a feeling, and you realize that your anger has much deeper roots than you thought ... ... But even if you haven't recognized what it's really about, you can be sure that the old feelings of inferiority and with them the anger are dissolving ... ... because you are now closer to yourself than before, and your inner helper is sending you thoughts and feelings that gradually penetrate you and help you to recognize ... ... and with recognition, you free yourself ... ... Then your helper places a hand on your heart, and you feel the old pain slowly dissolve ... ... The painful feelings disappear because your helper takes them from you ... ... He/She will bring these feelings to the place of experience, and there they will remain as memories ... ... But you will be free, and you will be open to new and positive experiences ... ...

... ... Your inner helper says goodbye and goes to your inner center, because there your inner helper is always ... ... and so it should happen every day ... ... again and again ... ... because this helper is always and everywhere available to you ... ... He/She is a part of you ... ... As soon as you wake up in the morning and your day begins, you automatically encounter this helper and thus yourself ... ... deep in your feeling ... ... deep inside you, in your inner center, you encounter yourself ... ... the helping and experienced part of you, who also helped you today ... ... and again and again, this experienced and loving part helps you process your experiences ... ... for you and with you together ... ... for a good feeling ... ... for freedom and lightness ... ... for openness and even for joy of life ... ... for you ... ...

Hypnosis 7

… … You have experienced offenses and humiliations that made you angry and grumpy … … You know it's possible to let go of the anger … … You also know that now is the right time to let go of all feelings of offense and humiliation … … and more than that … … You can even do something in case you experience such feelings again … … to then let go of them again and again in peace … … You can build new self-confidence, a new and strong sense of self-worth with this letting go … … You can truly build this new attitude of strength … …

… … In your inner center, you now find a place of deep calm … … in your inner center, you always find a place of deep calm … … The calm of your body helps you feel and find this place within you … … The more clearly you can feel the calm of your body now, very consciously, the faster it becomes completely calm and still inside you … … The more you succeed in fully embracing the calm, the faster it becomes really calm and still inside you … … the faster you feel your inner center ... ... You feel your inner center ... ... Now ... ...

... ... And in the stillness of the inner center, you hear healing words ... ... You can hear them clearly ... ... Words that you let sink in deeply for your liberation ... ... for letting go of anger and resentment ... ...

+++ Variant 1: Anger, General +++

... ... I accept my story in peace and turn to others with new openness and kindness ... ...

+++ End of Variant 1 +++

+++ Variant 2: Anger as Self-Aggression +++

... ... I accept my story as it was, and I love myself as free as I now am ... ...

+++ End of Variant 2 +++

... {Please read the affirmations a bit slower and louder than the rest of the text and pause for 5-10 seconds after the affirmation before continuing to read!} ...

... ... Now feel the effect of these words ... ... their constructive effect spreads if you allow it ... ... that's already enough ... ... Simply allow these special words to spread their constructive effect ... ... so it is good ... ... very good ... ...

... ... Now consciously feel the closeness to yourself ... ... feel the closeness to your feelings ... ... to your moods and emotions ... ... You are close to yourself ... ... now ... ... so it is good ... ... very good ... ...

... ... Your subconscious stores the words as your affirmation ... ... as your deep belief ... ... as your new inner truth ... ... as an inner truth that also becomes outer truth ... ... so it is good ... ... very good ... ...

... ... Now feel how from your innermost being ... ... deep within yourself ... ... a new truth emerges ... ... through the effect of your special affirmation ... ... and feel that every repetition of your affirmation reinforces its helping effect ... ... now and whenever you hear it ... ... or speak it ... ... or think it ... ... so it is good ... ... very good ... ... Your affirmation is the affirmation, the confirmation and reinforcement of your new truth ... ... so it is good ... ... very good ... ...

... ... Every conscious and intense repetition of your affirmation renews and reinforces the constructive effect ... ... Deep inside, you say once again, and again and again ... ...

+++ Variant 1: Anger, General +++

... ... I accept my story in peace and turn to others with new openness and kindness ... ...

+++ End of Variant 1 +++

+++ Variant 2: Anger as Self-Aggression +++

... ... I accept my story as it was, and I love myself as free as I now am ... ...

+++ End of Variant 2 +++

... ... and now enjoy the relaxation of the trance you are in ... ... Trust in the unfolding of the optimal and helping effect of the affirmation for you, because it will happen ... ... today and every other day ... ... because you have succeeded in accepting the affirmation and really feeling it ... ... feeling that it belongs to you ... ... feeling that it is good and right ... ...

... ... So good ... ... You have achieved a lot ... ... You have now changed your attitude with a simple and absolutely powerful affirmation ... ... You have accepted your very personal affirmation and deeply integrated it into your feeling ... ... as your attitude ... ... as your feeling ... ... as your truth ... ... And you can experience this new truth every day ... ... You can consciously and intentionally use your affirmation every day to further free yourself from resentment and anger ... ... to further optimize your liberation and realignment ... ... and it is easy to do ... ... In a conscious moment ... ... by turning to yourself and with mindfulness for your thoughts and feelings, you can keep repeating your affirmation ... ... or whispering it ... ... or thinking it ... ... and thus further reinforce the positive effect ... ... freeing yourself again and again from old thought patterns and continuing on your constructive path ... ... every day ... ... really every day ... ...

Hypnosis 8

… … You have dealt with your anger and have realized that it stands in your way … … You've understood that this deep anger, this resentment, has no causes in the present but arose from the interaction of many painful experiences … … In the past, all of this arose, so you want to give it back to the past … … Today, you can speak with an instance that can truly help you overcome the anger … … Perhaps you are religious and can pray … … to God or to Jesus or to an angel … … or you speak with yourself because you believe there is a power deep within you that can and will help you … … your subconscious or your inner reflection … … Decide for yourself with whom you want to speak, but you are always speaking with an important and strong part of yourself … … with a part that listens to you and supports you … … You might say … …

Neutralization … … Dear Me in the Mirror / Dear God / Dear Guardian Angel / Dear Subconscious … … I have understood that I must overcome my anger … … I know that it is old disappointments and humiliations that make me feel a fundamental anger and often become angry or harsh without reason ... ... I know that there were many events and situations where I felt inferior and had to endure them, which I didn't handle well ... ... But all that was in the past and should remain in the past ... ... Dear Me in the Mirror / Dear God / Dear Guardian Angel / Dear Subconscious ... ... I ask for your help so that I can truly give the past back to the past and always remind myself that my life today has nothing to do with the past ... ... because only then will I be truly free from resentment and anger ... ... and I want to be free ... ... I really want to be free ... ...

+++ Variant 1: Anger, General +++

... ... Dear Me in the Mirror / Dear God / Dear Guardian Angel / Dear Subconscious ... ... I am fully aware that I must find trust again and give trust ... ... Only with trust can a happy and contented life be achieved ... ... I trust in your guidance and your help ... ... Yes, I trust that you ... ... dear Me in the Mirror / dear God / dear Guardian Angel / dear Subconscious ... ... can and want to help me ... ... and I also want to do my part and really try and let go ... ... I am fully aware that it takes my firm will to trust again, but I can do it … … I am sure I can do it, and with your support, I will really succeed … … I want that … … I really want to trust … … I really want to be calm and friendly … … I really want to be fair because I know that only in this way can I experience my daily life with an open mind and encounter my fellow human beings … …

+++ End of Variant 1 +++

+++ Variant 2: Anger as Self-Aggression +++

… … Dear Me in the Mirror / Dear God / Dear Guardian Angel / Dear Subconscious … … I am fully aware that I must also forgive myself … … Only with self-love can a happy and contented life be achieved … … I trust in your guidance and your help … … Yes, I trust that you … … dear Me in the Mirror / dear God / dear Guardian Angel / dear Subconscious … … can and want to help me … … and I also want to do my part and meet myself with consideration and openness … … I am fully aware that it takes my firm will to allow self-love again, but I can do it … … I am sure I can do it, and with your support, I will really succeed … … I want that …

... I really want to accept and love myself ... ... I want to meet myself again freely and openly ...

+++ End of Variant 2 +++

... ... Dear Me in the Mirror / Dear God / Dear Guardian Angel / Dear Subconscious ... ... I know that I must first overcome my fear ... ... my fear of being disappointed and humiliated ... ... I am ready for that ... ... With your help and with your support ... ... dear Me in the Mirror / dear God / dear Guardian Angel / dear Subconscious ... ... I will succeed ... ... I also know that I must take care of all my feelings ... ... I want and I will accept all my feelings and recognize them as my own, even the pressure behind the anger, because that way, I can also let it go ... ... It is important to accept my feelings as my inner experience and thus be able to let go of the feelings ... ... and I want to do that with your help ... ... dear Me in the Mirror / dear God / dear Guardian Angel / dear Subconscious ... ... from today on, again and again ... ...

... ... Dear Me in the Mirror / Dear God / Dear Guardian Angel / Dear Subconscious ... ... Please also help me to stay strong if I can't let go of the anger as quickly as I actually want to ... ... that I continue to believe that I can let go and overcome resentment and anger over time ... ... I know I must be patient with myself ... ... Maybe my inner self needs some time to completely overcome the old pain and the resulting anger ... ... then I want to give myself that time too ... ... I thank you now for your support ... ... dear Me in the Mirror / dear God / dear Guardian Angel / dear Subconscious ... ...

... ... Good ... ... Now allow yourself to enjoy the peace a little longer and just be here, because now you don't have to do anything more ... ... Everything important has already been done ... ... Now the support of your helper becomes support within you ... ... help from you for you ... ... So, you can trust in double help ... ... So, your deepest inner self is set to do everything that helps you overcome and finally let go of the old anger and build new trust and self-love ... ... Trust and self-love that you can give again ... ... your trust ... ... your self-love ... ...

Hypnosis 9

… … Today, you may deal with your deep feelings … … because you finally want to let go of your deep bitterness and all thoughts of revenge … …

… … Today, you may find peace within yourself … … because you finally want to let go of your deep bitterness and all thoughts of revenge … …

… … Today, you may overcome old anger and hatred … … because you finally want to let go of your deep bitterness and all thoughts of revenge … …

… … Today, you may end your self-blame and self-accusation … … because you finally want to let go of your deep bitterness and all thoughts of revenge … …

… … Now focus on the beautiful moments in life … … and that's why the deep anger is also dissolving more and more, and inner peace is setting in … …

…… You know that what has already happened cannot be changed …… and that's why the deep anger is also dissolving more and more, and inner peace is setting in ……

…… You know that the end of thoughts of revenge frees you …… and that's why the deep anger is also dissolving more and more, and inner peace is setting in ……

…… You can and you may live in peace with yourself …… and that's why the deep anger is also dissolving more and more, and inner peace is setting in ……

…… You recognize and feel inner peace again in the depth of your feelings ……

…… Feel the relaxation of your body and let it become emotional relaxation …… because with this feeling, you can also let go of thoughts of revenge ……

…… Feel the well-being of your body in this moment …… because with this feeling, you can also let go of thoughts of revenge ……

…… You feel that physical and inner calm are healing …… because with this feeling, you can also let go of thoughts of revenge ……

... ... Trust your body, which shows you that letting go of anger frees you ... ... and with this feeling, you can also let go of thoughts of revenge ... ...

... ... You recognize and feel inner peace again in the depth of your feelings ... ...

... ... Now, in the calm of trance, you also feel pleasant feelings within you again ... ... That helps you overcome and let go of deep resentment ... ...

... ... Now, in the calm of trance, you also feel new lightness again ... ... That helps you overcome and let go of deep resentment ... ...

... ... Now, in the calm of trance, you also feel new freedom again ... ... That helps you overcome and let go of deep resentment ... ...

... ... Now, in the calm of trance, I feel the closeness to myself ... ... That helps you overcome and let go of deep resentment ... ...

... ... You recognize and feel inner peace again in the depth of your feelings ... ...

+++ Variant 1: Anger, General +++

… … Take some time every day for reflection and mindfulness … … so you feel peaceful moods and feelings again that are good for you … …

… … Really look forward and enjoy new encounters … … so you feel peaceful moods and feelings again that are good for you … …

… … Go through everyday life consciously and attentively every day … … so you feel peaceful moods and feelings again that are good for you … …

… … Forgive yourself for what you once blamed yourself for … … so you feel peaceful moods and feelings again that are good for you … …

… … You recognize and feel inner peace again in the depth of your feelings … …

+++ End of Variant 1 +++

+++ Variant 2: Anger as Self-Aggression +++

… … Take some time every day for reflection and mindfulness … … and with mindfulness and self-respect, you meet yourself every day … …

… … Really look forward and enjoy new encounters … … and with mindfulness and self-respect, you meet yourself every day … …

… … Go through everyday life consciously and attentively every day … … and with mindfulness and self-respect, you meet yourself every day … …

… … Forgive yourself for what you once blamed yourself for … … and with mindfulness and self-respect, you meet yourself every day … …

… … You recognize and feel inner peace again in the depth of your feelings … …

+++ End of Variant 2 +++

… … It is clear to you, of course, that reconciliation primarily means reconciliation with yourself … … that's why you stay on your personal path of peace with and to yourself … …

…… It is also clear to you that letting go of anger and overcoming thoughts of revenge have already freed you today …… that's why you stay on your personal path of peace with and to yourself ……

…… You know exactly that you are on your way …… on your personal path of peace …… that's why you stay on your way …… Yes, you stay on your way ……

Hypnosis 10

... ... You know the constant resentment and bitterness ... ... You've felt these feelings and this mood for so long, and often you don't even know exactly why ... ... You've certainly had to endure some blows in your life and have experienced some defeats or humiliations ... ... Some things may have gone unprocessed and are still deep inside you as disappointment or offense ... ... So, it may have happened that you are angry and bitter ... ...and often feel this quiet resentment ... ... You just haven't really let it out yet ... ... have suppressed and repressed these feelings ... ... Maybe you also felt guilty too often and therefore didn't allow yourself your anger ... ... Over time, suppressed anger then became constant resentment ... ... But that's exactly what you want to end ... ... The good thing is that you don't have to find a specific cause for it ... ... You don't have to find what or why it happened, because there are always many causes together ... ... The path of letting go and liberation is much more important ... ... and for that, it is important that you free yourself from feelings of guilt ... ... that you can accept yourself ... ... can accept your story because you don't have any other ... ... Even if you think that you somehow made yourself guilty, even if you are very sure of it, now is the time to forgive yourself ... ... and if there are thoughts of revenge because you were wronged, then you can also let go of this desire for revenge because trapped in anger, you would only suffer for the injustice of others ... ... In the state of trance, your subconscious can really help you ... ... It is waiting for you to speak to it ... ... And that is easy today ... ... Just allow my words to become yours by saying ... ...

... ... I accept my past because it is the only one I have ... ...

... ... because I have recognized that everything in life truly has meaning ... ...

... ... {approx. 5-10 seconds of silence} ...

... ... I accept my past because it is the only one I have ... ...

... ... because I have recognized that only in acceptance can anger and resentment disappear ... ...

... ... {approx. 5-10 seconds of silence} ...

... ... I accept my past because it is the only one I have ...

... ... because I have recognized that feelings can never harm me ... ...

... ... {approx. 5-10 seconds of silence} ...

... ... I accept my past because it is the only one I have ...

... ... because I have recognized that in this way, I end my suffering ... ...

... ... {approx. 5-10 seconds of silence} ...

... ... I accept my past because it is the only one I have ...

... ... because I am worth it ... ... because I am truly worth it ... ...

... ... {approx. 5-10 seconds of silence} ...

+++ Variant 1: Anger, General +++

... ... I forgive myself for thoughts of revenge and retribution ... ...

… … because I have recognized that they were expressions of my inner distress … …

… … {approx. 5-10 seconds of silence} …

… … I forgive myself for thoughts of revenge and retribution … …

… … because I have recognized that my thoughts were like inner self-defense … …

… … {approx. 5-10 seconds of silence} …

… … I forgive myself for thoughts of revenge and retribution … …

… … because I have recognized that I can also be lenient with myself … …

… … {approx. 5-10 seconds of silence} …

… … I forgive myself for thoughts of revenge and retribution … …

… … because I have recognized that I am still a good person … …

… … {approx. 5-10 seconds of silence} …

... ... I forgive myself for thoughts of revenge and retribution ... ...

... ... because I am worth it ... ... because I am truly worth it ... ...

... ... {approx. 5-10 seconds of silence} ...

+++ End of Variant 1 +++

+++ Variant 2: Anger as Self-Aggression +++

... ... I forgive myself for the anger I had towards myself ...

... ... because I have recognized that it was primarily an expression of my despair ... ...

... ... {approx. 5-10 seconds of silence} ...

... ... I forgive myself for the anger I had towards myself ...

... ... because I have recognized that I was actually searching for self-love ... ...

... ... {approx. 5-10 seconds of silence} ...

… … I forgive myself for the anger I had towards myself …

… … because I have recognized that I no longer want to harm myself … …

… … {approx. 5-10 seconds of silence} …

… … I forgive myself for the anger I had towards myself …

… … because I have recognized that this feeling also belongs to my past … …

… … {approx. 5-10 seconds of silence} …

… … I forgive myself for the anger I had towards myself …

… … because I am worth it … … because I am truly worth it … …

… … {approx. 5-10 seconds of silence} …

+++ End of Variant 2 +++

… … I love myself with all my weaknesses and flaws … …

… … because I have recognized that in this, I find my peace … … {approx. 5-10 seconds of silence} …

… … I love myself with all my weaknesses and flaws … …

… … because I have recognized that I can always find the feeling of self-love deep within me … …

… … {approx. 5-10 seconds of silence} …

… … I love myself with all my weaknesses and flaws … …

… … because I have recognized that only then do I also receive more respect from the outside … …

… … {approx. 5-10 seconds of silence} …

… … I love myself with all my weaknesses and flaws … …

… … because I have recognized that in this way, I also honor and respect myself … …

… … {approx. 5-10 seconds of silence} …

… … I love myself with all my weaknesses and flaws … …

… … because I am worth it … … because I am truly worth it … …

… … {approx. 5-10 seconds of silence} …

Distribution, publication, and copying in any form are prohibited and subject to damages.

All Titles in the Series

Volume 1: Smoking Cessation
Volume 2: Anxiety and Restlessness
Volume 3: Burnout
Volume 4: Reducing Overweight
Volume 5: Coping with the Past
Volume 6: Suicidal Thoughts and Attempts
Volume 7: Psycho-Oncology
Volume 8: Obsessions and Tics
Volume 9: Self-Confidence and Decision-Making
Volume 10: Grief Work
Volume 11: Psychosomatics
Volume 12: Chronic Pain
Volume 13: Depressive Thoughts
Volume 14: Panic Attacks
Volume 15: Domestic Violence, Victim Support
Volume 16: Post-Traumatic Stress
Volume 17: Exam Anxiety and Stage Fright
Volume 18: Anti-Violence Training, Offender Support
Volume 19: Addiction Tendencies
Volume 20: Social Phobia and Fear of Contact
Volume 21: Nail Biting
Volume 22: Self-Awareness and Self-Love
Volume 23: Teeth Grinding and Night Clenching
Volume 24: Feelings of Guilt
Volume 25: Fear in Crowds
Volume 26: Fear of Flying, Aviophobia
Volume 27: Fear in Enclosed Spaces, Claustrophobia
Volume 28: Tinnitus, Ear Noises
Volume 29: Fear of Heights
Volume 30: Neurodermatitis

Copying, publishing, and sharing with third parties are only permitted with the written consent of the author. Please observe the notes on copyright and usage.

Volume 31: Finding Inner Balance
Volume 32: Overcoming Loneliness
Volume 33: Fear of Illness, Hypochondria
Volume 34: Anticipatory Anxiety, Fear of Fear
Volume 35: Jealousy in Relationships
Volume 36: Driving Anxiety
Volume 37: New Start after Separation
Volume 38: Fear of Injections
Volume 39: Heart Anxiety Neurosis
Volume 40: Overcoming Resentment and Anger
Volume 41: Resolving Blockages and Positive Thinking
Volume 42: Stress Reduction, Stress Management
Volume 43: Body Relaxation
Volume 44: Deep Relaxation
Volume 45: Fear of the Dark
Volume 46: Falling Asleep and Staying Asleep
Volume 47: Compulsive Buying
Volume 48: Restless Legs Syndrome
Volume 49: Bulimia
Volume 50: Anorexia
Volume 51: Overcoming Nightmares
Volume 52: Imagined Deformity
Volume 53: Overcoming Distrust, Finding Trust
Volume 54: Processing Failures
Volume 55: Humiliation, Emotional Hurt
Volume 56: Distressing Compassion, Vicarious Suffering
Volume 57: Self-Forgiveness
Volume 58: Self-Awareness, Self-Confidence
Volume 59: Saying No
Volume 60: Assertiveness
Volume 61: Setting Boundaries and Self-Assertion
Volume 62: Decision-Making Ability

Volume 63: Success Orientation
Volume 64: Ruminating, Circular Thinking
Volume 65: Accepting Pregnancy
Volume 66: Birth Preparation
Volume 67: Spiritual Opening
Volume 68: Joy of Life and Inner Lightness
Volume 69: Patience and Inner Peace
Volume 70: Fibromyalgia and Rheumatism
Volume 71: Irritable Bowel Syndrome, Crohn's Disease
Volume 72: Fear of Nausea, Emetophobia
Volume 73: Stuttering and Cluttering, Speech Flow Disorders
Volume 74: Concentration and Knowledge Anchoring
Volume 75: Vitality and Spontaneity
Volume 76: Searching for Meaning and Finding Goals
Volume 77: Life Crises, Life Events
Volume 78: Workaholism, Goal Obsession
Volume 79: Helper Syndrome, Helpless Helpers
Volume 80: Medication Abuse
Volume 81: Gambling Addiction
Volume 82: Internet Addiction, Smartphone Addiction
Volume 83: Hoarding Disorder, Compulsive Collecting
Volume 84: Conspiracy Thoughts, Overvalued Ideas
Volume 85: Fear of Operations and Treatments
Volume 86: Fear of Aging
Volume 87: Travel Anxiety
Volume 88: Anxiety When Urinating, Paruresis
Volume 89: Fear of Intimacy and Togetherness
Volume 90: Fear of Blushing
Volume 91: Coming Out in Homosexuality
Volume 92: Charisma Training
Volume 93: Migraines and Chronic Headaches
Volume 94: Overcoming Allergies, Bronchial Asthma

Volume 95: Normalizing Blood Pressure
Volume 96: Compulsive Perfectionism
Volume 97: Sports Hypnosis, Motivation
Volume 98: Sports Hypnosis, Performance Enhancement
Volume 99: Determination and Focus
Volume 100: Encountering the Inner Child
Volume 101: Cravings, Binge Eating
Volume 102: Stimulating Metabolism
Volume 103: Bipolar Mood Swings
Volume 104: Borderline, Identity Crises
Volume 105: Hypomania, Euphoria, Mania
Volume 106: Restlessness, Agitation
Volume 107: Nervous Breakdown
Volume 108: Adjustment Disorders
Volume 109: Self-Alienation, Depersonalization
Volume 110: Ending Self-Pity
Volume 111: Primary Gain of Illness
Volume 112: Secondary Gain of Illness
Volume 113: Bullying, Victim Support
Volume 114: Letting Go of Envy and Jealousy
Volume 115: Fear of Spiders, Arachnophobia
Volume 116: Fear of Dogs or Cats
Volume 117: Fear of Strangers, Xenophobia
Volume 118: Excessive Worries, Generalized Anxiety
Volume 119: Strengthening Sense of Responsibility
Volume 120: Unrequited Love, Heartache
Volume 121: Work-Life Balance
Volume 122: Letting Go of Unattainable Goals
Volume 123: Allowing and Accepting Help
Volume 124: Letting Go of Adult Children
Volume 125: Tourette Syndrome
Volume 126: Life Changes and New Starts

Volume 127: Accepting Life in a Wheelchair
Volume 128: Understanding and Overcoming Homesickness
Volume 129: Understanding and Overcoming Wanderlust
Volume 130: Dizziness, Meniere's Disease
Volume 131: Overcoming Aggression
Volume 132: Cutting and Self-Harm
Volume 133: Hair Pulling, Trichotillomania
Volume 134: Postpartum Depression
Volume 135: For Relatives of Dementia Patients
Volume 136: Self-Harm, Artificial Disorders
Volume 137: Activating Self-Healing Powers
Volume 138: Preventing Depression Relapse
Volume 139: Reactive Psychoses, Follow-Up
Volume 140: Obsessive Thoughts and Impulses
Volume 141: Compulsive Checking
Volume 142: Compulsive Counting, Symmetry Obsession
Volume 143: Compulsive Washing, Cleanliness Obsession
Volume 144: Compulsive Questioning
Volume 145: Dissociative Paralysis
Volume 146: Phantom Pain
Volume 147: Overcoming Complaining
Volume 148: Hay Fever, Pollen Allergy
Volume 149: Sexual Abuse, Victim Support
Volume 150: Standing Strong Against Sexism, #metoo
Volume 151: Binge Eating
Volume 152: Overcoming Thoughts of Revenge
Volume 153: Detachment from the Aggressor, Stockholm Syndrome
Volume 154: Courage to Separate
Volume 155: Chronic Fatigue, Exhaustion
Volume 156: Fear of the Future, Existential Anxiety
Volume 157: Excessive Worry About Children
Volume 158: Fear of Failure

Volume 159: Ending Distrust and Control
Volume 160: Dejection, Dysphoria
Volume 161: Boreout, Chronic Boredom
Volume 162: Bipolar Disorders, Relapse Prevention
Volume 163: Mania, Relapse Prevention
Volume 164: Nihilism, Feelings of Worthlessness
Volume 165: Thumb Sucking
Volume 166: Being Brave
Volume 167: Being Proud
Volume 168: Overcoming Shyness
Volume 169: Being Able to Delegate Responsibility
Volume 170: Being Able to Show Emotions
Volume 171: Letting Go of Guilt, Victim Support
Volume 172: Processing Guilt, Offender Support
Volume 173: Mood Swings, Cyclothymia
Volume 174: Lack of Drive, Vital Sadness
Volume 175: Hearing Voices with Reality Reference
Volume 176: Confident Communication
Volume 177: Standing Up for Oneself
Volume 178: Taking New Paths
Volume 179: Confident Job Application
Volume 180: No Longer Being Taken Advantage Of
Volume 181: End of Submissiveness
Volume 182: Depressive Numbness
Volume 183: Mood Drops, Affective Incontinence
Volume 184: Mood Instability
Volume 185: Somatoform Disorders
Volume 186: Stomach Ulcer, Psychosomatic
Volume 187: Accepting Amputation
Volume 188: Overcoming and Letting Go of Hatred
Volume 189: Ending Accusations
Volume 190: Allowing Tears, Being Able to Cry

Volume 191: Finding and Sorting Repressed Feelings
Volume 192: Somatoform Pain
Volume 193: Living Autonomously
Volume 194: Anhedonia, Joylessness
Volume 195: Persistent Sadness
Volume 196: Obesity, Food Addiction
Volume 197: Parents of Abused Children
Volume 198: Letting Go and Letting Be
Volume 199: Childhood Sexual Abuse
Volume 200: Fear of Loss

www.ingramcontent.com/pod-product-compliance
Lightning Source LLC
Chambersburg PA
CBHW030450220526

45464CB00006B/2473